DEADLY APOTHECARY ORACLE

Priestess Moon

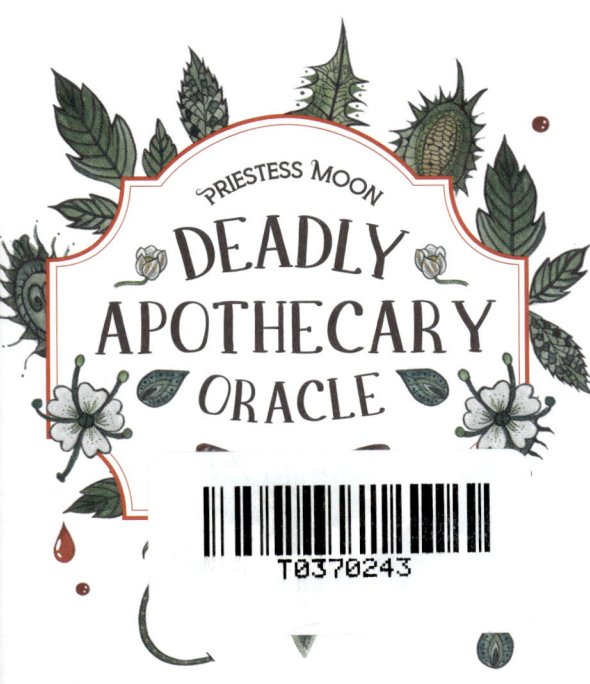

POISONOUS PLANTS AS GUIDES AND HEALERS

ROCKPOOL

A NOTE ON POISONOUS PLANTS
*In these modern times, these plants must not be
touched or consumed unless administered
by a trained practitioner.*

A Rockpool book
PO Box 252
Summer Hill
NSW 2130
Australia

rockpoolpublishing.com
Follow us! **f** 📷 rockpoolpublishing
Tag your images with #rockpoolpublishing

ISBN 9781922785664

Published in 2024 by Rockpool Publishing
Text and illustrations © Priestess Moon 2024
Copyright design © Rockpool Publishing 2024

Cover design by Sara Lindberg, Rockpool Publishing
Internal design and typesetting by Alissa Dinallo, Rockpool Publishing
Edited by Lisa Macken

Printed and bound in China
10 9 8 7 6 5 4 3 2 1

All rights reserved. No part of this publication may be reproduced,
stored in a retrieval system, or transmitted in any form or by any
means, electronic, mechanical, photocopying, recording or otherwise,
without the prior written permission of the publisher.

CONTENTS

INTRODUCTION	1
HOW TO USE THE CARDS	5
FIVE SIGNS THAT THE *DEADLY APOTHECARY ORACLE* IS WORKING	13
DEADLY APOTHECARY CARDS	15
1. Destroying Angel: soul contracts	16
2. Deathcap: step into your power	18
3. Hemlock Water-dropwort: trust that feeling	20
4. Black Hellebore: drop the drama	22
5. Angel's Trumpet: open your mind	24
6. Baneberry: just ask!	26
7. Lily of the Valley: open your heart	28
8. Arum Lily: courage of convictions	30
9. Snowdrop: go with the flow	32
10. Stinging Nettle: rethink restriction	34
11. Boggard Posy: gossip and kindness	36
12. Poison Ivy: psychic vampire	38
13. Thornapple: embrace your weirdness	40
14. Cuckoo-pint: sovereign boundaries	42
15. Cannabis: the healer	44
16. Mistletoe: interdependence	46
17. Giant Hogweed: in/tolerance	48
18. Fly Agaric: virtual reality	50

19. Foxglove: magickal thinking	52
20. Tobacco: the guru	54
21. Opium Poppy: share your light	56
22. Belladonna: accept your fate	58
23. Monkshood: witchcraft	60
24. Larkspur: bright star	62
25. Madonna Lily: spiritual superiority	64
26. Mandrake: obsession	66
27. Henbane: away with the fae	68
28. Black Bryony: catharsis	70
29. Narcissus: walk away	72
30. Nutmeg: manifesting	74
31. Castor Bean: release the past	76
32. Hemlock: psychic protection	78
33. Holly: allow wealth	80
34. Cherry Laurel: peacekeeper	82
35. Yew: embrace change	84
36. Liberty Cap: surrender	86

BIBLIOGRAPHY   **88**

ACKNOWLEDGEMENTS   **91**

ABOUT THE AUTHOR AND ILLUSTRATOR   **92**

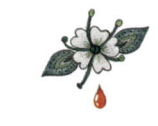

Introduction

All of the plants in this deck are considered to be toxic when touched or ingested, and some are even illegal. However, in just the right amounts they can be powerful medicines that heal and restore. It's all about getting the dosage right: the dose makes the poison. Many so-called deadly herbs are remarkable healers, similar to how we wouldn't have been born with the ability to feel negative emotions if they weren't valuable. Emotions that aren't positive are not bad or a sign of weakness; they are part of being human and living life on this earth school.

Divine Feminine

The Priestesses of Poison embody the spirit of each poisonous plant and represent a uniquely feminine energy. The divine feminine is the intuitive, nurturing, patient and wise energy that will help you as you journey with your shadow self. Think of this deck as an apothecary: while the cures may take work, the results will be worth it.

Instead of working on the physical level, the priestesses in this deck work with the devas of the plants on an energetic level. *Deva* means 'body of light' in Sanskrit and, thus, we are working on an etheric, not a physical, level with this plant magick oracle.

THE POISONS AND THE ANTIDOTES

While there are no reverse meanings in this deck, each card has a poison aspect and an antidote. The Priestesses of Poison each represent a character that embodies a particular behaviour.

The poisons: we come to earth to experience a full range of emotions, both good and bad. Every human engages in uncomfortable thoughts and behaviours, and everyone has a favourite go to for when they are feeling hurt or stressed – expressing anger, blame, playing the victim, being a drama queen, jealousy and so on. We harshly judge ourselves and others for these strong emotions, but it is one of the main reasons we are here experiencing life on earth in human form.

These behaviours are very necessary and helpful in showing you where you are not being true to yourself or whether your boundaries have been crossed. Your darkest aspects can also be your greatest teachers. If you stuff down emotions and pretend everything is fine you will remain stuck. It's a message for you to really examine these behaviours and why you engage in them time after time. To see the pattern is to break the pattern.

It's easy to fall into a good vibes only trap, thinking that to be a spiritual person you must be always happy and positive. The truth is that as a human you need to sit with your uncomfortable feelings and work out what their message is to you. Invalidating or minimising your emotions, always trying look on the bright side, ignoring crappy behaviours from others or glossing over painful feelings suppresses an important human experience. Being positive is a worthy trait, but if it comes at the expense of diminishing your very real lived experience or that of other people it becomes counterproductive.

The antidotes: your soul characteristics are the qualities that make life sweeter and help others. These are your awake actions, where you consider how we are all connected. Light emotions come from your heart and lead to beautiful synchronicities and joyful experiences. When you make decisions that align with your true nature you brighten your light and bring balance to your mind, body and spirit, which in turn helps others to brighten their light. You will need to journey through the dark often until you get to this light.

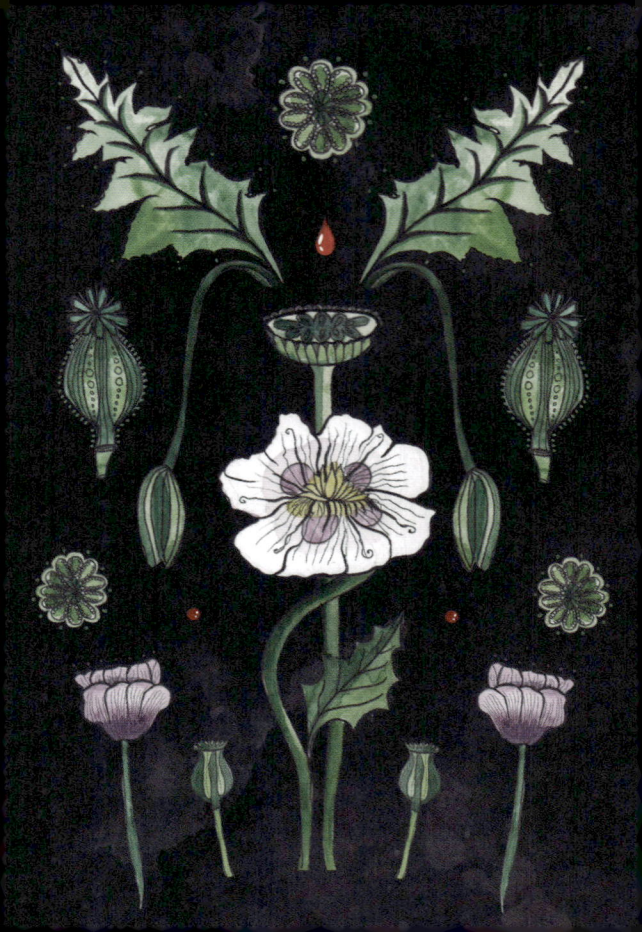

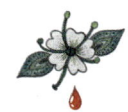

HOW TO USE THE CARDS

Each card represents a particular human behaviour or emotion. Every single card features a character, a Priestess of Poison represented by a plant. Each plant has a message for you that highlights the behaviour you are dealing with and brings with it a message of healing. Once you can clearly see how others have been treating you or how a belief or behaviour is doing yourself or others a disservice you can be aware of it, and this is the first step towards healing. This is all said without judgement. I can guarantee you that as the author of this deck I have experienced every single one of these behaviours and emotions!

You may resonate with the card meaning, or just the poison or antidote. Perhaps just one sentence in the guidebook will give you the insight you need, and this is enough. Discard the rest of if it doesn't ring true.

Before you work with the Priestesses of Poison, practise the following exercise to bless your deck and connect with your soul.

- Take three deep breaths and imagine there is a golden light in your heart that gets brighter with each breath.

- Ask your guides and angels to be present and that you be open to any insights.

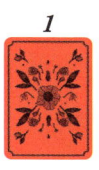

ATHAME LAYOUT

Cut through to the heart of the issue like a knife cutting through leaves and roots with this one-card spread. Shuffle the cards while asking a question, and choose just one card from the deck. You will see the behaviour featured in the card either in yourself or someone you are interacting with, and it will give you a good overview of the energies you're dealing with.

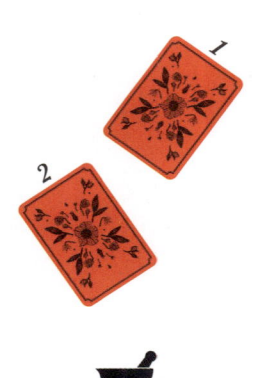

MORTAR AND PESTLE LAYOUT

Just as the pestle grinds plants in a mortar for healing cures, this layout grinds down to the crux of the problem. A two-card spread, the pestle (card 1) represents the person you are dealing with and the mortar (card 2) represents you. Shuffle the cards and choose two from the deck. With the first card the pestle will give you an insight into what the other person is feeling and thinking and how their behaviour is influencing you. With the second card the mortar will show you a behaviour of your own you may not have considered.

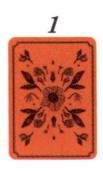

Personality preview

If you have ever wondered what someone else is thinking or what their motivation is for a certain behaviour, this deck can offer insight. Shuffle the cards, concentrating on the person and your interactions with them, then choose one card. There will be a certain type of character represented in the card, which will give you a good idea of where the person's behaviour is coming from, why they do what they do and how to better understand them.

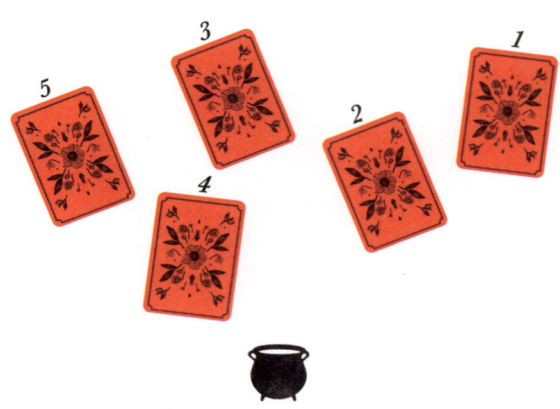

CAULDRON LAYOUT

Cauldrons are used to steep and cook herbs for potions and poultices, with many herbs combined to make a powerful healing draught. This five-card spread is a melting pot of ideas to consider, as humans are complex creatures who can feel many emotions at once. Shuffle the deck, choose five cards then look at the characters on each card to get a comprehensive snapshot of the situation. Each card can represent a different personality in a group of people, and it's fun to work out who is represented by each card. See how the behaviours/personalities combine to give you a broader overview of the energies and emotions at play.

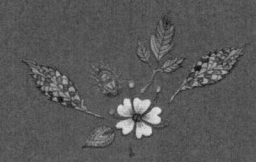

Dedicated to all who are challenged by life in human form on earth. It's easy to get caught up in the drama of our story and forget who we really are: limitless, shining souls.

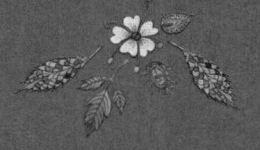

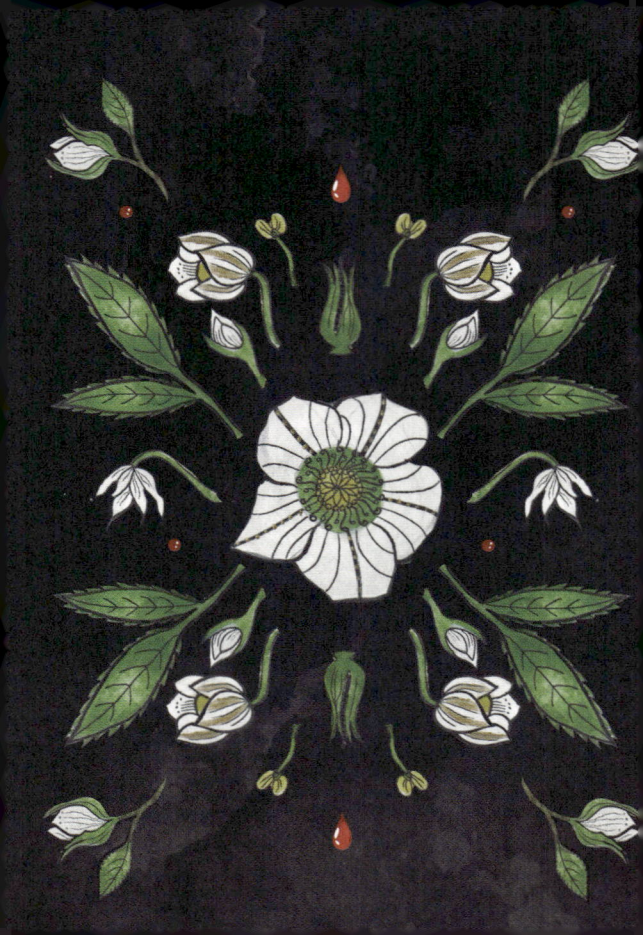

5

FIVE SIGNS THAT INDICATE THE *DEADLY APOTHECARY ORACLE* IS WORKING

1. You recognise the behaviours in yourself and others, feeling compassion for both.

2. You can laugh at these behaviours and see things from a higher perspective.

3. You are no longer so easily offended.

4. You acceptYL and identify negative emotions without shame and as part of your human experience.

5. You clearly express your needs and desires without having to resort to manipulative behaviours.

*For every human illness,
somewhere in the world there
exists a plant which is the cure.*

— Rudolph Steiner

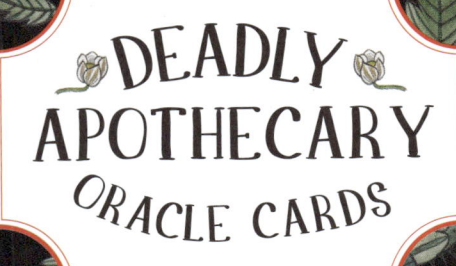

DEADLY APOTHECARY
ORACLE CARDS

1. Destroying Angel
Soul contracts

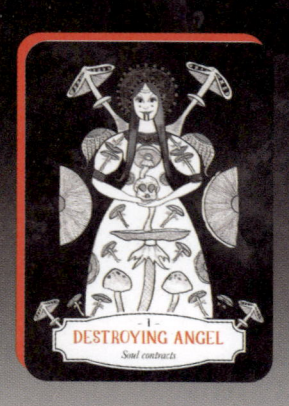

Botanical name: Amanita virosa.
Energy: detached and merciless.
Other names: European destroying angel amanita.
Traditional/medicinal uses: as with Deathcap (card 2),
Destroying Angel's medicinal potential
is being researched.
Magickal/historical uses: no known magickal uses.
No known antidote if ingested; it shows no mercy.

THE POISON

Destroying Angel has been wronged and is filled with a righteous wrath. They will stop at nothing to make sure that the person who has crossed them will suffer. Like an avenging angel, they are consumed with fury and will give no quarter; however, the punishment they seek outweighs the crime. They are not thinking rationally, and deliberately go out of their way to hurt someone. Onlookers can understand why they feel this way but are starting to wonder if Destroying Angel has taken it too far.

THE ANTIDOTE

There's a reason why Destroying Angel's enemy has stirred up so much emotion: they are soul bound and were contracted to meet and challenge each other before they incarnated on earth. By putting so much energy into retribution, Destroying Angel's bond to their nemesis becomes stronger and more constrictive. For them to end the connection they can visualise ripping up the soul contract and saying: 'I release you. We are no longer bound. Our contract is null and void.' They will find that the ire will dissipate and they will start to dissociate from their enemy. While the actions of their enemy are never condoned, the hold over Destroying Angel will be lessened and they will, at last, find peace.

2. DEATHCAP
Step into your power

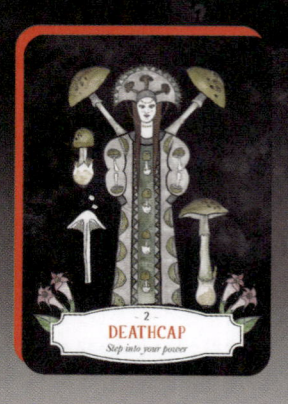

Botanical name: Amanita phalloides.
Energy: deadly, cloaking and dark.
Other names: deadly amanita.
Traditional/medicinal uses: it is the subject of research for medicinal potential.
Magickal/historical uses: no known magickal uses.

THE POISON

Deathcap has been taught to be quiet from an early age, shutting down powerful emotions again and again to make life easier for those around them. Deathcap was often silenced. They learned to be meek and not cause too much trouble, realising their strong and sensitive feelings were an inconvenience and would not be tolerated. To please others Deathcap became obedient and passive, trying very hard not to make any waves. They have repressed their strong feelings for so long they are starting to feel numb and powerless.

THE ANTIDOTE

Deathcap has forgotten they are a powerful being, temporarily dulled by living in human form. They believed too much in what others said about them and have been overly dutiful and timid, which has clouded their light. Deathcap needs to step into their power and realise that their sensitivity is their strength. Their strong feelings are now safe to express, which will lead to powerful changes for themselves and the world. It is time for Deathcap to realise their strength and start by expressing their needs and wishes in relationships.

3. HEMLOCK WATER-DROPWORT
Trust that feeling

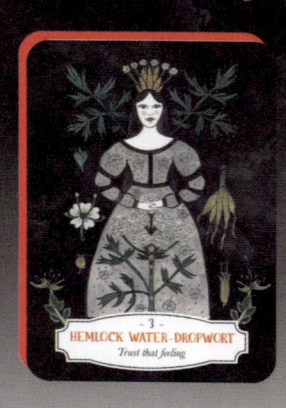

Botanical name: Oenanthe crocata.
Energy: quick, virulent and startling.
Other names: dead man's fingers, water-hemlock.
Traditional/medicinal uses: it was used in poultices to clean wounds but it is not employed in modern medicine.
Magickal/historical uses: no known magickal uses. A popular poison in ancient times, it affects the facial muscles and leaves its victims with a startling grin often called a 'sardonic smile'.

THE POISON

A sardonic grin is a smile that never travels to the eyes; therefore, not everything is as it seems. Dropwort hides behind a seemingly innocuous facade, but once you scratch the surface things can get ugly. Dropwort wears a mask of niceness and faux concern that leaves you wondering why you feel uncomfortable in Dropwort's presence despite the pleasant character. Could it be because they are saying lovely things, socially acceptable things, while all the time wishing you ill with their thoughts?

THE ANTIDOTE

Discernment is so important when you interact with characters such as Dropwort. Do not rely on Dropwort's words and how they present themselves. Instead, rely on how they make you feel. If you walk away feeling exhausted after Dropwort has been love bombing you then alarm bells should be ringing. Even if the logical conclusion says they have your best interests at heart or you still feel uneasy, learn to trust that feeling for it will always steer you right. Dropwort's games do not need to be played.

4. BLACK HELLEBORE
Drop the drama

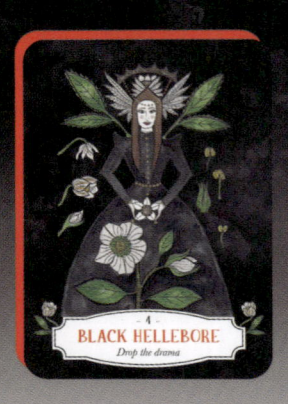

Botanical name: Helleborus niger.
Energy: narcotic, mystic and pure.
Other names: Christ herb, Christmas rose, melampode.
Traditional/medicinal uses: the black root was dried and powdered to treat hysteria and calm strong emotions.
Magickal/historical uses: in folk magic, casting the powdered root into the air was thought to render a person invisible.

THE POISON

For Hellebore strong emotions act like a narcotic: they are addicted to the drama. Hellebore lurches from self-created crisis to crisis, never really enjoying peace and calm. They centre themselves in every tragedy, enjoying the attention, and are dependent on powerful emotions to make them feel energised. If life is getting a bit dull and quiet, Hellebore will create a commotion just so they can feel alive again.

THE ANTIDOTE

Intense emotions are something we have been gifted with to help us focus on what we want to manifest. The heady feeling of strong emotions can be addictive, and is one of our huge lessons on earth. Do not confuse passion and intensity with aliveness when these strong feelings are used to feed a habit and garner attention. Hellebore can drop the drama this time around.

5. ANGEL'S TRUMPET
Open your mind

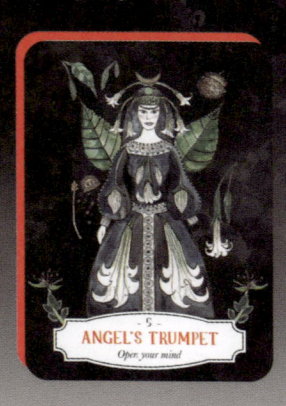

Botanical name: Brugmansia suaveolens.
Energy: flighty and ethereal.
Other names: angel's tears.
Traditional/medicinal uses: it was used in ointments as a pain reliever and anti-inflammatory.
Magickal/historical uses: it symbolically represents the resurrection and life after death. In ancient times it was used in rituals for its euphoric and hallucinogenic properties to contact spirits.

THE POISON

Angel has closed their mind and believes only in what they can see, hear and touch; things must be scientifically proven before given any credibility. Angel smirks when people bring up subjects such as life after death or communication with spirits because they are highly sceptical of any spiritual nonsense and believe this makes them a very intelligent and logical person. A little scepticism is healthy; outright cynicism is not. Angel shields their mind to delicious possibilities when all they really need to do is trust and open their mind to new ways of thinking.

THE ANTIDOTE

The human body is a vehicle that we drive while on this planet. It houses the eternal soul, which continues to live on once the human host dies. This is not false hope: the survival of consciousness after physical death is close to being scientifically proven with inventions such as the SoulPhone. Angel can be open to the idea that life goes on even when the physical body doesn't. They will awaken to this knowledge when the time is right, and it will bring them much peace and understanding.

6. BANEBERRY
Just ask!

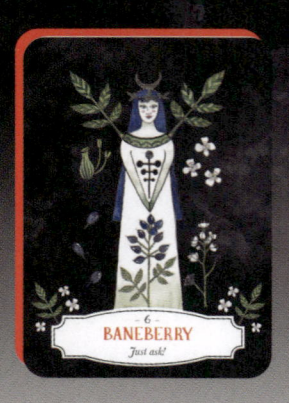

Botanical name: Actaea spicata.
Energy: lurking, concealed and expelling.
Other names: bugbane, herb Christopher, toadroot.
Traditional/medicinal uses: the root has been used in folk remedies to treat headaches, coughs, colds and joint inflammation. The berries are extremely poisonous when ingested but can be used to make a rich, black dye when crushed and macerated.
Magickal/historical uses: it can be used in binding spells. The plant has a peculiar, odious smell that is very attractive to toads.

THE POISON

Baneberry has seen bossy and demanding people get their own way and does not like this behaviour, so they will act meek and compliant to feel superior. They will nod and smile and say everything is okay when asked but later complain about not being considered. They will also sneakily go behind people's backs to get their way. Baneberry is quite manipulative and doesn't like asking for what they want outright. They conceal their needs and desires by hinting and indirect questioning, but all they really need to do is just ask!

THE ANTIDOTE

It's true that being bossy and demanding isn't nice, but neither is it good to be meek and sneaky. This plant medicine is a lesson in speaking up and not hiding your wants and needs. Baneberry is allowed to state what they want and would like. We all are but then we let it go, knowing that we have stated our case and that our preferences have been heard and may be considered. Baneberry has expressed and been true to themselves, and in the end this is what really matters.

7. Lily of the Valley
Open your heart

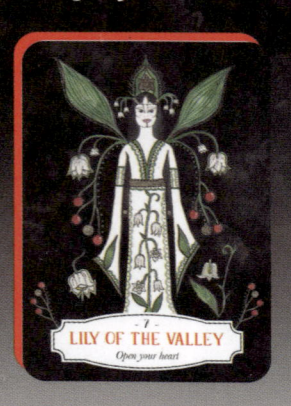

Botanical name: Convallaria majalis.
Energy: comforting, heady and perfumed.
Other names: Jacob's ladder, our lady's tears.
Traditional/medicinal uses: the plant was used in medicines to treat weak hearts; however, the active compound is now manufactured in a laboratory.
Magickal/historical uses: it is often used in love spells. It's known for its ephemeral nature, because once picked it will last just one day.

THE POISON

Lily has closed their heart. They no longer want to get close to others, because they know they will just end up being hurt. Lily knows that nothing lasts and feels that the pain of losing someone is not worth the love they have invested. Lily has convinced themselves that being alone is best, so they push people away and will not pursue relationships even though this will bring them much joy.

THE ANTIDOTE

Love is all there is. The nature of life on earth is ephemeral and nothing lasts forever, which is one of the hardest lessons to learn. We are here to make connections with others, and while they may not last in the physical world we will see each other again in the spirit world. Those we have loved and lost will be there, waiting for us when it is our turn to leave this earthly realm. Even those who have hurt us we will make amends with, and the joy of connection will be felt once again. Once Lily realises this they will find a beautiful world of emotional riches waiting for them.

8. Arum Lily
Courage of convictions

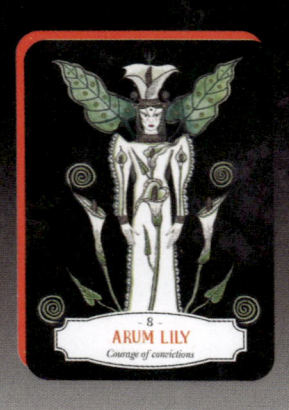

Botanical name: Zantedeschia aethiopica.
Energy: glowing, snowy and smooth.
Other names: calla lily, green goddess.
Traditional/medicinal uses: the tubers were used as a South African folk remedy to topically treat wounds. They should never be ingested.
Magickal/historical uses: they are used in spells to connect with the power of the divine feminine. They flourish quickly and are extremely resilient.

THE POISON

The disempowered Arum lives in doubt and fear. They are constantly worried about what others will think of them or if they are doing the right thing. They are scared of being judged, cancelled and shut down for their beliefs. As a result, Arum does nothing and remains stuck, their beautiful gifts to humanity languishing and becoming atrophied. They need to practise their resilience by fully believing in themselves and standing up to the naysayers with power and grace. Arum needs to have the courage of their convictions.

THE ANTIDOTE

Once Arum has tapped into their resilience and power, watch out: there is no stopping them! Beautiful, heart-centred determination and a willingness to make the world a better place become their life mission. They embody goddess energy, knowing who they are and that they are on earth to make a difference – and they will.

9. SNOWDROP
Go with the flow

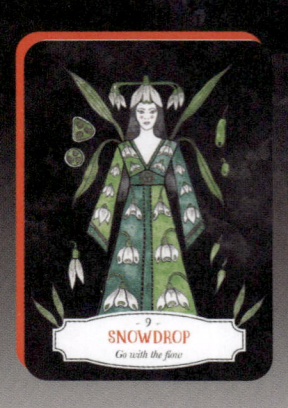

Botanical name: Galanthus nivalis.
Energy: opening and stimulating.
Other names: fair maid of February.
Traditional/medicinal uses: it contains a substance called galanthamine, which has been proven useful in managing certain forms of dementia.
Magickal/historical uses: the first flower to appear after winter, they herald the return of light and warmth and are a symbol of rebirth and the triumph of light over dark.

THE POISON

Snowdrop has a hard time accepting the cycles of life. When things are going well they worry that something bad will happen. When things are going badly they think the good times will never arrive again. Snowdrop is stuck in a pessimistic thought frequency and always expects the worst to happen. They focus on the negative and forget to be grateful for what they already have.

THE ANTIDOTE

It's the nature of life to have its ups and downs, and the best way for Snowdrop to deal with this is to pretend that life is a river and they are a leaf just going with the flow. Sometimes the way will be rocky and difficult and other times it will be plain sailing. Release the need to control outside influences and go with the flow of life's journey. Snowdrop can listen to the whispers of their guardian angel. It's all part of the polarities of life on earth – the opposites, the good and the bad: one cannot be appreciated without the other. Enjoy the good times, and when the bad times come know they will not last and the light will come back into life.

10. STINGING NETTLE
Rethink restriction

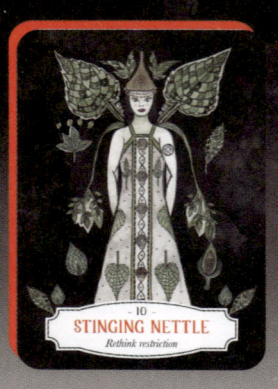

Botanical name: Urtica dioica.
Energy: verdant and nurturing.
Other names: common nettle, lesser nettle.
Traditional/medicinal uses: the juice makes a fortifying tonic that helps with gout, anemia and kidney problems.
Magickal/historical uses: they are used in spells for protection and fertility. Nettles are nutritionally dense plants that can be used to make delicious soups, beers and wines.

THE POISON

Stinging Nettle has decided to cut a few things from their diet in a bid to become healthier. It all starts innocently enough: for the first few weeks their willpower is strong, and it's going so well they decide to restrict a few more items. Then the restriction becomes a game to see how long they can stretch the time between meals. Stinging Nettle's world becomes a narrow focus of restraint and never quite feeling full enough, but they think about food all the time. Meals out with family and friends become joyless tasks filled with anxiety, because restriction has led to obsession.

THE ANTIDOTE

The human body is such a clever machine, knowing intuitively when and what to eat and when to stop. Taste buds become dulled once the stomach registers fullness. Restrictive diets don't give long-term results, and constraint and control around food steals joy and comes at too high a price. Stinging Nettle can rethink restriction and relax into the idea that their body knows best, and if they let it guide them then hunger and fullness become second nature. Weight doesn't necessarily correlate to health. One of the delightful things about having a corporeal body is the full enjoyment of food and drink while on earth.

II. BOGGARD POSY
Gossip and kindness

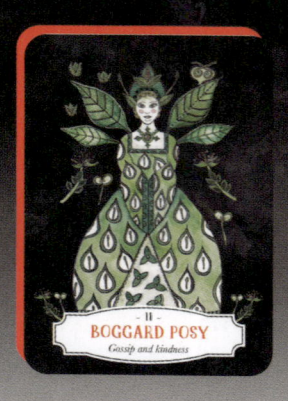

Botanical name: Mercurialis perennis.
Energy: warty, wary and acrid.
Other names: dog's mercury.
Traditional/medicinal uses: the leaves were mixed with vinegar and sugar to cure warts.
Magickal/historical uses: can be used in spells to dispel gossip. In English folklore a boggard is a cheeky house spirit that enjoys causing trouble and likes to scrape a slimy hand across people's faces while they sleep.

THE POISON

Boggard Posy loves a good gossip. Most of us do: humans are sociable creatures and are hard wired to be curious about their neighbours' and friends' lives. As Jane Austen once wrote: 'For what do we live, but to make sport for our neighbours, and laugh at them in our turn?' However, Boggard Posy takes it too far, embellishing and speculating for attention and shock value. They get carried away and forget to be kind. Be wary of any information about another person you hear from Boggard Posy as it may be pure fiction.

THE ANTIDOTE

When Boggard Posy discusses their feelings one on one with a friend about how others have treated them it is not gossip, it's a healing means to work out their boundaries with certain people. However, if they are in a group and hear something detrimental about someone else they must ask themselves if the news is helpful and true or just scurrilous speculation? Boggard Posy is best to adopt an attitude of kindness and think twice before they pass on gossip or spread misinformation. Words have power, so make them kind and beautiful when you speak about others.

12. POISON IVY
Psychic vampire

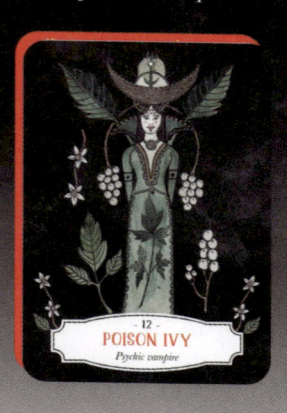

Botanical name: Toxicodendron radicans.
Energy: creeping, blistering and tranquilising.
Other names: eastern poison ivy, poison vine.
Traditional/medicinal uses: in homeopathy it is deemed to be a good remedy for sprains and arthritis.
Magickal/historical uses: it holds a very protective energy and can be used in spells for blocking unwanted interactions with others.

THE POISON

The disempowered Poison Ivy is an energy or psychic vampire and a bit of a taker in friendships. They like useful friends and often ask for favours without returning them but they seem to have forgotten that friendship is a two-way street. They are the kind of friend who will only appear when they want something. Poison Ivy is very good at one-sided conversations, often becoming quite emotional and demanding comfort and mutual outrage, but the recipient of these strong emotions might not have the capacity to deal with the onslaught and feels uncomfortable. It's difficult, as Poison Ivy has had a challenging life and deserves compassion.

THE ANTIDOTE

Friendship is a mutual relationship built on respect and reciprocation. If Poison Ivy shifts the focus away from themselves for a moment they may realise that their friends also need help and support. The give and take of friendship is highlighted. When Poison Ivy needs to rant they can ask their friend first if they are in the right emotional space to listen to them. Instead of constantly dumping on others, they can speak to a trusted therapist or record their upset in a journal, as this can help to process strong emotions.

13. THORNAPPLE
Embrace your weirdness

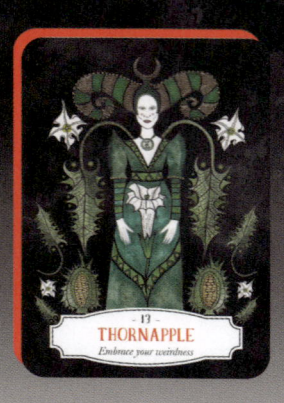

Botanical name: Datura stramonium.
Energy: unique, powerful and hallucinogenic.
Other names: datura, devil's trumpet, jimsonweed.
Traditional/medicinal uses: in some folk remedies ointment of thornapple was used topically to alleviate inflammation of all kinds.
Magickal/historical uses: in ancient times priestesses and oracles ingested the plant to help aid their prophetic visions. Its striking appearance is unmistakable and cannot be confused with others.

THE POISON

Thornapple stands out from the crowd and is very self-conscious about it. Their appearance is unusual in some way, and they tend to dress drably so they don't draw attention. They have distinctive ideas and ways of dealing with life that others just don't appreciate and often feel misunderstood. They would love to express themselves more creatively through dress and fashion but are worried they will be ridiculed further.

THE ANTIDOTE

Thornapple was never meant to blend in: their soul purposely chose to be a peacock in this lifetime. Once they embrace this and start expressing themselves fully then, in time, they will realise their unique take on life will bring joy to themselves and others. We are not meant to be carbon copies of each other, all dressing, looking and thinking the same. Thornapple was always meant to think outside the box and express themselves with outlandish outfits and ideas. When Thornapple embraces their weirdness they pave the way for others to also express themselves in beautifully distinctive ways.

14. CUCKOO-PINT
Sovereign boundaries

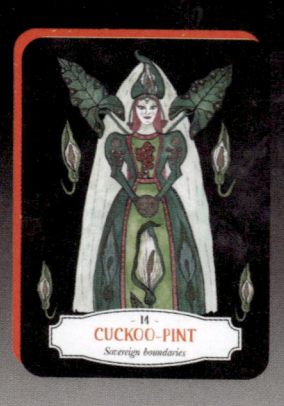

Botanical name: Arum maculatum.
Energy: striking and restorative.
Other names: arum, lords and ladies, wake robin.
Traditional/medicinal uses: the dried root was mixed with honey and taken as a stimulant for those exhausted by sickness.
Magickal/historical uses: the metaphysical properties include the balancing of masculine and feminine energies and ensuring harmonious relationships.

🌿 THE POISON 🌿

Cuckoo-pint has no boundaries in personal relationships. In romantic relationships they want so much to make their partners happy that they lose themselves in the union and often get burned. They have an access all hours vibe about them and tend to attract the takers. In friendships, Cuckoo-pint offers to help even though they are exhausted and are giving from an empty cup. They automatically say 'Yes' without thinking things through and always regret it when the time comes to honour that 'Yes.'

🌿 THE ANTIDOTE 🌿

Cuckoo-pint is allowed to say 'No': access to their precious energy should be treated like a golden ticket! They can practise setting some sovereign boundaries with others and learn not to over-commit their precious time. The next time they are asked for a favour they can pause and reflect on whether it will be good for them or not and answer accordingly. The restorative nature of Cuckoo-pint asks you to fill your own cup with delightful activities that make you happy and brighten your own light before you offer your valuable time and energy to others.

15. CANNABIS
The healer

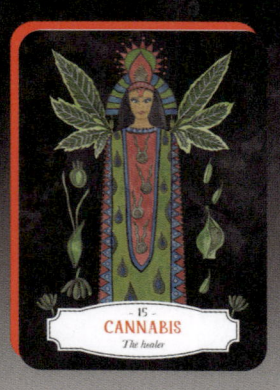

Botanical name: Cannabis sativa.
Energy: healing and dreamlike.
Other names: bhang, ganja, hemp, marijuana, weed.
Traditional/medicinal uses: it is used medicinally to help aid sleep and reduce physical pain.
Magickal/historical uses: in ritual settings it can be smoked to produce prophetic visions and receive messages from the spirit realm. When used inappropriately it will cause paranoia and demotivation.

THE POISON

The disempowered Cannabis is easily overwhelmed and suspicious of everyone, the mindset of which is partly because they have a habit of playing the victim. They are stuck in childhood wounds and tend to overreact to many things, citing a painful past. Prone to self-pity and asking 'Why me?', Cannabis believes the world owes them a living. They give their power away by too often identifying with their human ego and forget that they are a limitless, shining spirit.

THE ANTIDOTE

Cannabis has the potential to become a powerful healer once they have completed their shadow work, but for now they are stuck in habitual responses like a recording on repeat. They can do the following things with intention, which will start the healing process: shine a light on all the yucky stuff such as the shadows so they may be brought to the surface to be healed; stop defining themselves by their past and release the wounds from childhood; and understand that they and they alone are responsible for their life. These processes will release Cannabis from feeling overwhelmed and usher them into a new way of being as a healer.

16. Mistletoe
Interdependence

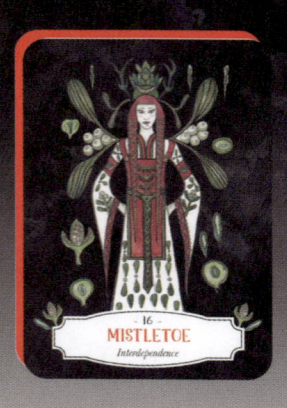

Botanical name: Viscum album.
Energy: strengthening and fortifying.
Other names: herbe de la Croix, lignum crucis, mystyldene.
Traditional/medicinal uses: in 17th-century herbals a tonic of the leaves and twigs was suggested to calm the nerves and muscles and help in the treatment of epilepsy and headaches.
Magickal/historical uses: it is a sacred plant of the Druids said to banish evil and bring in good blessings for the new year. It is a parasite yet it forms a symbiotic relationship with its host plant.

THE POISON

Mistletoe is fiercely independent. They do not rely on anyone else for anything and are proud of being a self-made person. They believe that asking for help is a sign of weakness, and can often be heard saying: 'If you want something done right, you have to do it yourself.' Mistletoe will not turn to others for assistance even when they need it, for they have learned to be strong and trust only themselves.

THE ANTIDOTE

Having the confidence and self-belief to be an independent person is an admirable trait but this plant medicine highlights hyper-independence; that is, when a person will not accept help from anyone even though they need it. The truth is that we are all *inter*dependent, we are all connected and are meant to help and heal each other. No one can be truly independent. Mistletoe should understand that many hands have worked together to bring them their food, clothes and shelter, that they haven't done every single thing themselves and they don't need to.

17. Giant Hogweed
In/tolerance

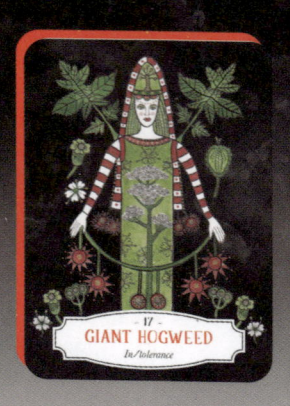

Botanical name: Heracleum mantegazzianum.
Energy: looming, scorching and strange.
Other names: giant cow parsley or parsnip, hogsbane.
Traditional/medicinal uses: some folk remedies use a decoction of the seeds to treat shingles and skin conditions.
Magickal/historical uses: it can be employed in healing and restorative spells and is a plant that will quickly control the environment it is in.

THE POISON

Hogweed is intolerant of other people's views and ways of doing things. They are loud and imposing and quickly take control in every situation. In fact, they are known as a bit of a control freak among friends and family, and are always trying to make sure things are taking place according to their rigid expectations. Tolerance is not their strong point. Hogweed will impose their desires on others to make sure everything goes their way.

THE ANTIDOTE

Hogweed can remind themselves that the following things are within their control: how they treat themselves and others; their thoughts and behaviours; and how they choose to spend their time. Everything else is out of their personal control, so they can surrender the need for micromanagement and ask their higher self for the strength to be tolerant and compassionate, allowing others to sometimes be in charge.

18. Fly Agaric
Virtual reality

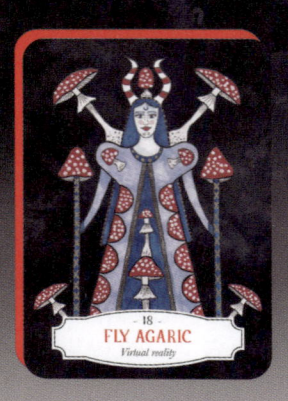

Botanical name: Amanita muscaria.
Energy: enchanting, playful and psychedelic.
Other names: fly amanita.
Traditional/medicinal uses: used in Eastern Europe and parts of Russia as an anti-inflammatory and pain reliever. Preliminary research suggests it might be useful to combat cognitive decline.
Magickal/historical uses: its distinctive red and white form is associated with fairies and magic. In past times it was used by Siberian shamans to produce hallucinations and visions of the future to help their tribespeople.

THE POISON

Fly Agaric sees the world differently to most people and doesn't get caught up in the expected norms of society such as having a full-time job, fancy house or car or social status, which baffles people. They realise that they have chosen to be human in what is essentially a virtual reality and refuse to play the game. However, so many are tied to their human story and they take the game very seriously. Fly Agaric does not seem to live in the real world, moving to the beat of their own drum, and this frustrates people who are playing the game.

THE ANTIDOTE

Fly Agaric is an expert in observation and going with the flow because they realised early on that many things are out of their control. They are always prepared to play and have a wicked sense of humour, and their company is much sought after. They have mastered the art of surrendering, allowing and watching with detached compassion as the world's dramas play out. They seldom get involved in dramas, trusting that everything that happens is for their highest good. Fly Agaric is an evolved soul who knows that this world is just an illusion, and they take great delight in living as their higher self.

19. FOXGLOVE
Magickal thinking

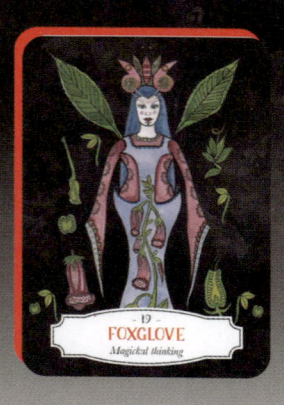

Botanical name: Digitalis purpurea.
Energy: strengthening, flowing and fluid.
Other names: dead men's bells, fairy caps, witches' gloves, lady's glove.
Traditional/medicinal uses: it is still used today in heart medications for irregular heartbeats and fluid build-up. Legend says it can raise the dead and kill the living.
Magickal/historical uses: it has long been associated with the faery folk because its preferred habitat is deep in forest glens where faeries reside. Spellcrafters can work with the energy of the plant to contact the fae.

🌿 THE POISON 🌿

The disempowered Foxglove has unrealistic expectations of themselves and others, who they believe should read their mind and automatically know what they want and need. They hold idealistic views about how things should be and think the world must fit this vision. Being optimistic is a good trait, but it's impossible to control everything and everyone with their magickal thinking! Every human is born with free will, which keeps things interesting. Unfortunately, when Foxglove's expectations are not met and usually by circumstances beyond their control they spiral into anger and frustration, becoming highly distressed and believing the world to be a very unkind place.

🌿 THE ANTIDOTE 🌿

There is nothing wrong with engaging in magical thinking from time to time; in fact, it can help spark optimism and lighten the heart. However, it becomes a problem for Foxglove when it starts to affect everyday life and the belief they are in control of everything that happens. Unhelpful superstitions can lead to excess worrying and an overburden of assumed responsibility. One way Foxglove can live in this world with grace and ease is to lower their expectations. As Adi Da Samraj said: 'Relax, nothing is under control.'

20. TOBACCO
The guru

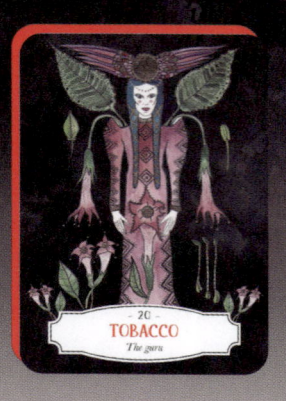

Botanical name: Nicotiana tabacum.
Energy: majestic, detoxifying and cleansing
Other names: tabacca.
Traditional/medicinal uses: fresh and dried leaves are thought to ward off disease because of their anti-fungal and anti-bacterial qualities.
Magickal/historical uses: its smoke is used to clear negative energy. It has been smoked in rituals since ancient times to visit alternate realities and contact those in the spirit world. The plant is seen as a great, healing spirit that should be treated with respect.

THE POISON

The disempowered Tobacco is attracted to religions and spiritual pursuits, not for insights and growth but for attention, adoration and the money to be made. They are quite cynical and know that people are easily influenced, and they exploit this. They have not studied at the feet of others but are a self-styled guru, a self-proclaimed shaman and a cultural appropriator of all things money making. Tobacco relies on their good looks and charm to lure people into their charlatan cult and fulfil their human desires in the name of spirituality.

THE ANTIDOTE

To check whether a spiritual teacher is teaching from universal love you check everything they say through the heart. A true guru does not incite fear or distrust, doesn't give doomsday prophecies for the future and doesn't proclaim that their teachings are the one and only. Genuine mentors teach only love and acceptance and are not motivated by great wealth. An empowered Tobacco is a true leader with humility, knowledge and compassion for the human experience who trusts in their guides and angels for the betterment of humanity. They receive and share great insights from ascended masters and use plant medicine respectfully.

21. Opium Poppy
Share your light

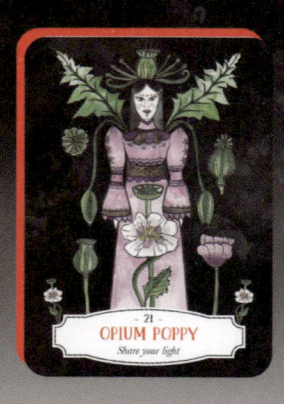

Botanical name: Papaver somniferum.
Energy: sedating and escaping.
Other names: breadseed poppy.
Traditional/medicinal uses: the narcotic sap has a hypnotic and sedative effect and is used to calm emotional and physical pain. Derivatives include morphine, codeine and heroin.
Magickal/historical uses: it is known to induce fantastical creative visions and spark innovative ideas. Spellworkers can work with the energy of the plant to manifest new ways of seeing things.

THE POISON

Opium Poppy dislikes interacting with others and will avoid them as much as possible because human behaviour and social norms baffle them. They choose not to partake in normal relationship milestones such as teenage romances, marriage and children. Unconsciously, they are choosing to remain alone and insular to consolidate their energy. They prefer their own world, with little disturbance from outside influences.

THE ANTIDOTE

Unbeknown to them and due to the amnesia we all endure as part of our human existence, Opium Poppy has incarnated on earth with a sacred mission. Their soul is from the stars and their purpose is to raise the energy of this planet, which they do by interacting with others and sharing their light. They must learn to be more generous with their time and energy. The main thing for them to remember is before they go to sleep at night they should release any energy that isn't theirs with deep outward breaths and call their own light energy back to them after each inward breath. In this way they will remain balanced.

22. BELLADONNA
Accept your fate

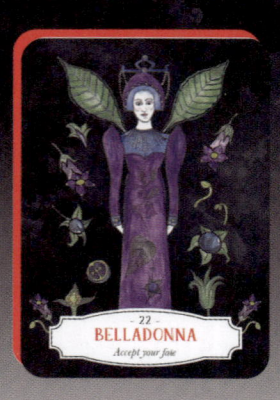

Botanical name: Atropa belladonna.
Energy: fated, sedated and glamorous.
Other names: deadly nightshade, devil's cherries.
Traditional/medicinal uses: used in the treatment of eye diseases and as a powerful muscle relaxant. Its sedating effect makes people seem unaffected by strong emotion.
Magickal/historical uses: it is associated with Atropos, one of the three Greek Fates who preside over human life. 'Bella donna' is Italian for 'beautiful woman'; its energy is perfect for glamour and beauty spells.

THE POISON

Belladonna has a bad habit of running away from accountability and escaping into a dream. To cope with difficult feelings and situations they procrastinate by putting off simple tasks and flaking out on responsibilities. They like to remain chill by adopting a good vibes only approach to life, minimising their pain and that of others. Anything that provokes strong and uncomfortable emotions will be deftly dodged by Belladonna. They expect people to be always love and light.

THE ANTIDOTE

It may seem counterintuitive, but the best way for Belladonna to work through an uncomfortable emotion is to feel it, really feel it, and not avoid it. Once they express that emotion fully they will be surprised at how quickly it passes. They must accept their fate as an emotional being and allow others to express their messy and uncomfortable emotions. After all, this is what we are here to learn about: to shine our light even when the world feels so dark. Holding space for others and facing our responsibilities becomes a joy when our emotions are clear.

23. MONKSHOOD
Witchcraft

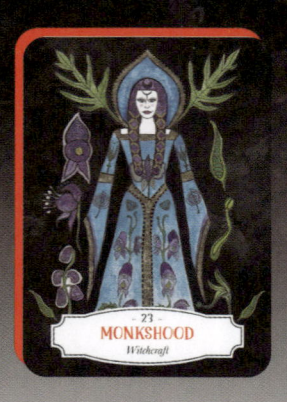

Botanical name: Aconitum napellus.
Energy: poisonous, pernicious and paralysing.
Other names: aconite, devil's bane, queen of poison, Venus's chariot, wolfsbane.
Traditional/medicinal uses: in folk remedies it was used to create a soothing topical salve for muscle and nerve pain.
Magickal/historical uses: it is so called because its strange flowers resemble the hood of a mediaeval monk's cloak. It is associated with Hekate, the goddess of witchcraft and magick.

THE POISON

The uncomfortable emotions Monkshood highlights are loneliness and censure: it brings up feelings of not belonging, of being victimised, misrepresented and misunderstood. Monkshood carries memories of a time when witches were burned at the stake for possessing powerful secret knowledge, for being too other. Associated with The Hermit card in tarot, it portends a time of solitude and reflection.

THE ANTIDOTE

Monkshood must hide away from the maddening crowd to rest, decompress and recharge. They can use this insular time to go deep within and find out who they truly are. While leaning into the nature of a hermit, monk, wise woman or witch it is the perfect time to focus on study, self-development and connecting to the higher self. This is slow time, crystalline, icy and wintery. The judgements of others do not matter; it is the perception of yourself that matters. Monkshood knows in their heart who they are and that their actions are pure.

24. LARKSPUR
Bright star

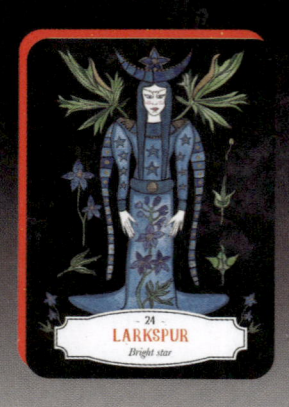

Botanical name: Consolida regalis.
Energy: wild, inky and cathartic.
Other names: field larkspur, lark's claw, knight's spur.
Traditional/medicinal uses: anecdotally, the juice of the leaves and flowers can help heal wounds.
Magickal/historical uses: it grows wild in the fields of Europe and can be employed in protection spells. Its beautiful bluish-purple, star-shaped flowers signify joy and a pure heart.

THE POISON

Larkspur had a difficult childhood, never really fitting in, and was branded as being weird and other and thus became a loner. They can never comprehend the violence and unkindness in the dense physical energy that is the earth, why people treat each other and the environment so badly. Larkspur has become insular, loathe to go out into the world and show who they truly are. They have forgotten they came here to help humanity, not to hide from it.

THE ANTIDOTE

The earth's energies are speeding up and changes are inevitable, and with this comes turbulence and uncertainty. Larkspur agreed to incarnate upon earth at this challenging time to help and heal humanity and guide them into a more peaceful, prosperous era. They have come from a place of unconditional love, creativity and joy; just their energy brightens a room. Larkspur must remember what they came here for and shine their light unapologetically, like a bright star in the sky.

25. Madonna Lily
Spiritual superiority

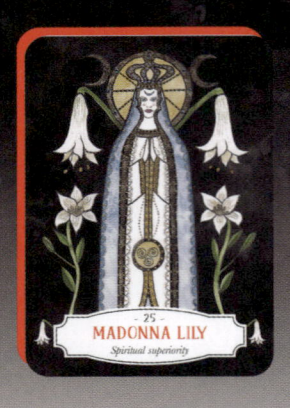

Botanical name: Lilium candidum.
Energy: perfect, pure and mystical.
Other names: lily of the field, white lily.
Traditional/medicinal uses: the bulbs were used in folk remedies to create a poultice for burns and ulcers and to heal bruises and skin conditions.
Magickal/historical uses: it is dedicated to Mother Mary, and through this association it has come to symbolise purity and innocence.

THE POISON

Madonna Lily is a very spiritual person – or at least they like to think so. They believe their diet and lifestyle is very clean and pure: they eat the right foods, practise the right exercises and spiritual ideals and generally think they have got it right. Unfortunately, all this righteousness comes with a large side order of judgment. With an air of imperiousness about them, Madonna Lily feels spiritually superior to those they consider unevolved. They allow ego to be in charge, feeling they are better than most people. A disempowered Madonna Lily has the personality of a disapproving mother superior.

THE ANTIDOTE

It's very human to judge and feel superior to others, but it's the opposite to what the soul feels. Ironically, feeling more spiritually advanced than others highlights lower-vibrational thoughts. The soul knows that we are all equal, that each soul is whole and complete and is a bright shining light that has chosen to experience life in human form on earth for a while.

We are all just trying to do our best in this challenging earth school. An empowered Madonna Lily helps people feel good about themselves no matter what stage of the evolutionary journey they are on.

26. Mandrake
Obsession

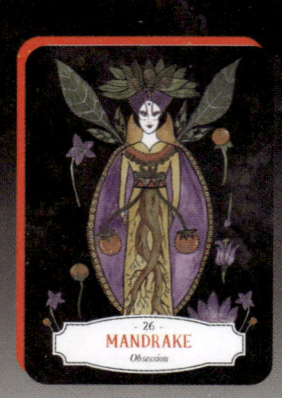

Botanical name: Mandragora officinarum.
Energy: intense and possessive.
Other names: Satan's apple, mandragora.
Traditional/medicinal uses: the root was used to create a sleeping draught for those in physical pain.
Magickal/historical uses: it's an hallucinogenic and key ingredient in witches' flying ointment, and was also a popular herb for love spells and considered an aphrodisiac. It was used in magickal rituals to drive away evil spirits.

THE POISON

Mandrake finds the feeling of falling in love intoxicating and gets bored when things become stable. They are obsessed with the first flush of a new relationship and will seek a dopamine hit time and time again, quickly discarding lovers and friends in search of the new, shiny and different. It's understandable they want to replicate that delicious feeling many times, but it comes at a huge cost to the well-being of the people in their destructive path and, eventually, to their own well-being. They will never, ever be satisfied.

THE ANTIDOTE

Mandrake is advised to spend some time alone, because the constant distraction of intense relationships bypasses the important work of getting to know themselves. Once they know who they truly are and what they truly want they will stop lurching from one meaningless relationship to the next and start focusing on what really matters to them. Obsessions will fall away, and inner peace will settle in.

27. HENBANE
Away with the fae

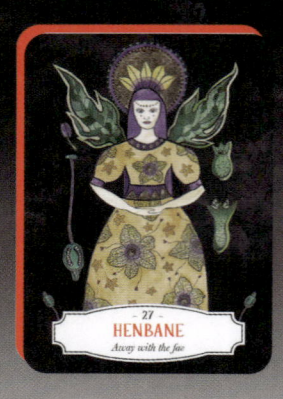

Botanical name: Hyoscyamus niger.
Energy: soporific and hypnotic.
Other names: black henbane, hog's bean, stinking nightshade.
Traditional/medicinal uses: it was used in folk remedies to treat headaches. The plant is used in modern medicine to treat epilepsy and Parkinson's disease.
Magickal/historical uses: during festivals the dried leaves were once added to beer for an extra narcotic kick so drinkers could really escape from the rigours of reality.

THE POISON

Henbane doesn't mean to be strange, but the normal rules of reality don't seem to apply to them. They have their feet firmly planted in mid-air and are often described as being away with the fairies. They live in their own little world, unaware of the effect they have on others. Their eyes are slightly glazed and they are hard to reach. Henbane will not be enticed to partake in the everyday, preferring escapism and being lost in dreams.

THE ANTIDOTE

We are all here on earth for a reason, experiencing life in human form in the here and now. Henbane can connect with others and come back to earth by grounding themselves, because life is so much sweeter and much more fun if you participate fully! By picturing a golden cord running from their solar plexus into the molten core of the earth they can start to remember who they are and why they are here. They can be wholly present, awake and aware and joyfully connecting with others.

28. BLACK BRYONY
Catharsis

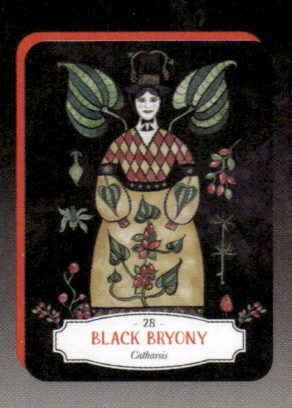

Botanical name: **Tamus communis** or **Dioscorea communis**.
Energy: irritating and purging.
Other names: blackeye root, black bindweed, lady's seal.
Traditional/medicinal uses: the fresh root was applied topically in folk medicine as a poultice, as it quickly disappears bruises and inflammation.
Magickal/historical uses: in magickal spells it is used to banish negative energy, purge the stale, old and unuseful and bring in the new.

THE POISON

Bryony feels powerless and unable to express their anger safely. They wear a friendly expression on their face but something is simmering behind the eyes, and they anger easily but hide it quickly. They have learned to control their anger by stuffing it down, holding it in and ignoring it; however, the anger will eventually creep up on them and express itself in weird ways such as a strange outburst, overreaction, baffling crying or an unexplained rash.

THE ANTIDOTE

The presence of anger is a pure gift that shows us there are deeper issues at play. Rage shines a spotlight on past hurts that have been left unresolved and on strong feelings that uncover important personal boundaries that have been crossed too many times. Black Bryony can meditate and go within to discover what these past hurts and personal boundaries are and why they are so important. Once the answers have been uncovered and their anger safely expressed the healing can begin. This process is beautifully cathartic.

29. NARCISSUS
Walk away

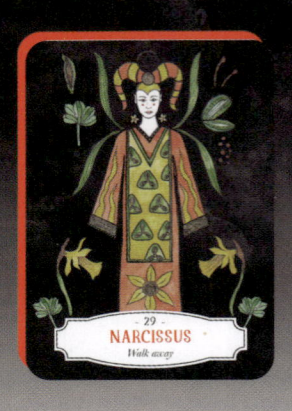

Botanical name: Narcissus pseudonarcissus.
Energy: gilded and banishing.
Other names: wild daffodil, Lent lily.
Traditional/medicinal uses: modern medical studies focus on the compound galantamine, which helps slow the progression of Alzheimer's disease.
Magickal/historical uses: it is excellent for use in love and money spells because of its sunny golden colour. However, take great care as the beautiful flowers hide poisonous bulbs.

THE POISON

When Narcissus is accused of emotionally hurting someone they deftly turn it around so they instead become the injured party. In the end it just becomes easier not to hold Narcissus accountable, allowing them to get away with spiteful behaviours again and again. At best the Narcissus character simply cannot see the points of view of other people and therefore lacks empathy, and at worst they find upsetting others a fun sport and will intentionally see if they can push people's buttons to get a reaction. They thrive on excluding others and creating toxic cliques.

THE ANTIDOTE

Narcissus is a glamorous character who is fun to be around until they turn on you, which they inevitably will. They love being chased and then find joy in rejecting those who are the keenest for their company. When you come across them and they ignore or avoid you, walk away. Don't seek to please them, chase their company or play their game out of some misplaced loyalty. Staying with someone for spiritual reasons or believing you can change them is an exercise in futility. Seek relationships and friendships where you are celebrated and feel included and supported, as this accepting energy will raise your frequency and help you enjoy more peaceful interactions with others.

30. NUTMEG
Manifesting

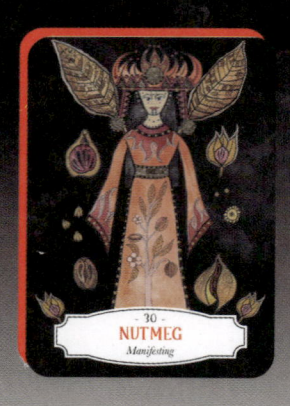

Botanical name: Myristica fragrans.
Energy: warming and comforting.
Other names: myristica, mace, true nutmeg.
Traditional/medicinal uses: it is often used in tonics to soothe digestive issues, and in sweet and savoury dishes to add a hint of comforting spice and roundness of flavour. However, if too much is ingested it can cause nausea and hallucinations.
Magickal/historical uses: it is employed in spells to manifest wealth and abundance.

THE POISON

In a disempowered state Nutmeg feels like a hapless victim to the vagaries of a capricious universe. They give their power away often, believing they have little control over their life. In an effort to gain some control they try law of attraction concepts by dreaming of a luxury car, social status, designer clothes and winning the lottery, but nothing seems to come to fruition.

THE ANTIDOTE

There is a shift in focus required away from immediate human longings to the desires of the soul while in this lifetime. Nutmeg focuses too much on human wishes and must realise that manifesting the life they want works best if it aligns with their soul's plan. It is easier to manifest opportunities than money or luxury items, so if Nutmeg concentrates on creating an ideal life by following and acting on their spiritual goals their life will transform. They can regularly check in with their soul to see if their manifesting is aligning with their higher good.

31. CASTOR BEAN
Release the past

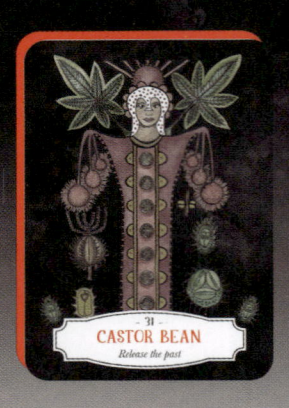

Botanical name: Ricinus communis.
Energy: slippery and cathartic.
Other names: castor oil plant, palma christi.
Traditional/medicinal uses: made from the seeds, castor oil is a well-known laxative because of its purgative nature. When applied topically it can help heal skin conditions.
Magickal/historical uses: the oil is used in spells to repel negative vibes and banish bad habits.

🌿 THE POISON 🌿

Castor Bean obsesses about the past, focusing on how things used to be instead of concentrating on the here and now. Prone to wistfulness, they believe that things were better back then, remembering only the good times, and have a tendency to hoard physical items. They often put past lovers on a pedestal. This behaviour causes pain for their current and future partners, who believe that if only they exhibited the same qualities Castor Bean would love them more. Castor is beholden to the long ago.

🌿 THE ANTIDOTE 🌿

It is draining being in a relationship with an emotionally unavailable person whose head is stuck in bygone days. It's not anyone's sole responsibility to make someone happy, especially those infatuated with the ghosts of the past. Castor Bean obsessing about what could or might have been has become a life stealer and they need to release the past. The universe works in mysterious ways, and if Castor Bean was truly meant to be with someone they would be. There can be no other way.

32. HEMLOCK
Psychic protection

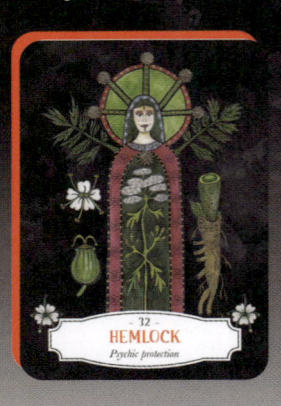

Botanical name: Conium maculatum.
Energy: hypnotic and pacifying.
Other names: herb bennet, poison hemlock, poison parsley, spotted hemlock, warlock's weed.
Traditional/medicinal uses: although extremely poisonous, in ancient times it was carefully prepared as a sedative for the nerves.
Magickal/historical uses: long associated with witches and witchcraft, it is a herb sacred to the goddess of witches Hekate. It is used in spells for protection and purifying.

THE POISON

Hemlock feels emotionally drained and physically exhausted after work and social interactions, often suffering from migraines. They leave themselves open to physical and spiritual energy vampires, as these individuals are attracted to their bright and open energy. The disempowered Hemlock lives in fear. They have dabbled with contacting the spirit world, but unfortunately did not prepare themselves properly and left their thoughts open to lower entities that thrive upon an anxious and worried mind.

THE ANTIDOTE

Before beginning any psychic work Hemlock can call upon Archangel Michael for protection. By imagining being bathed in a beam of electric blue light from this powerful angel they can burn away the detritus of human worries and feel the calmness of their soul taking charge. As an antidote to their exhausting social interactions they can imagine a beautiful bright bubble of white light around them and call in their guides and angels as a light shield throughout the day.

33. HOLLY
Allow wealth

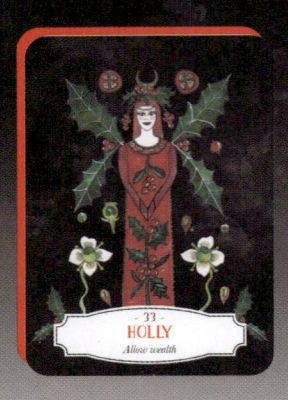

Botanical name: Ilex aquifolium.
Energy: glossy, crimson and spiked.
Other names: common holly, holm, holy tree, Christ's thorn.
Traditional/medicinal uses: the leaves have been used to treat fevers, jaundice and broken bones in the form of tinctures and poultices. Its poison reputation comes from the berries, which are violently purgative.
Magickal/historical uses: associated with the winter solstice and the festival of Yule, it is an evergreen that symbolises new life. If brought into the home during winter it brings wealth and good luck.

THE POISON

The disempowered Holly is jealous of the good fortune of others. They like to judge other people's spending habits on nice things or lavish holidays, often stating these people would be better off donating to charity. They become very envious and deeply feel the lack of indulgence in their own life, choosing to be offended by displays of wealth – which makes them very unhappy. There's nothing wrong with Holly wanting good fortune and comfort for themselves, but their poisonous behaviour demeans others for the enjoyment of wealth. They feel righteous when they disapprove of other people's prosperity, which makes them feel better about their own feelings of lack.

THE ANTIDOTE

Holly can give themselves permission to enjoy little luxuries without breaking the bank. They can accept that having money does not make you a bad person but instead adds to the enjoyment of life and helps others. They must realise that other people's finances are none of their business and concentrate on their own wealth. Rejoicing in the good fortune of others and imagining prosperity for themselves opens channels for receiving. Holly deserves more and can practise allowing more.

34. CHERRY LAUREL
Peacekeeper

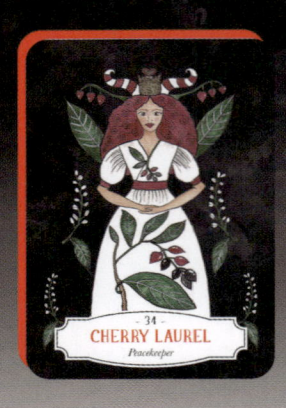

Botanical name: Prunus laurocerasus.
Energy: bitter and crystalline.
Other names: English laurel, common laurel.
Traditional/medicinal uses: it was used as a sedative to bring relief from insomnia and night coughs. The poisonous parts of the plants are the leaves, which contain small amounts of the deadly hydrocyanic acid.
Magickal/historical uses: the tree is used in protection and love spells.

THE POISON

The disempowered Cherry Laurel tries to keep the peace at all costs. If someone is upset they believe it is their personal responsibility to calm things down and make them right.

They avoid confrontation and are always the first one to yield, which leads to them being taken advantage of. Their feelings do not appear to matter, getting brushed aside and eclipsed by louder and more aggressive personalities. Cherry Laurel feels as though they are walking on eggshells with someone, which affects their health.

THE ANTIDOTE

Cherry Laurel has a natural calming energy, which makes them an ideal peacekeeper: a useful skill. However, they constantly misuse this ability by capitulating to a loved one. They can feel bitterness creeping in because their needs are always being ignored. Cherry Laurel is allowed to speak up and tell others if they feel they are being mistreated, even if this disturbs the peace and causes conflict. In fact, it is sometimes necessary. They say 'Choose your battles', and in this case Cherry Laurel must fight.

35. YEW
Embrace change

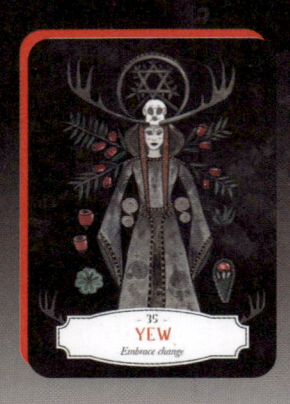

Botanical name: Taxus baccata.
Energy: hallowed and resurrecting.
Other names: common yew, English yew.
Traditional/medicinal uses: it is used in some homeopathic remedies.
Magickal/historical uses: it is a sacred Druidical tree and a symbol of life after death. A storm once upended an ancient yew tree in an English churchyard, and the next day entwined within its exposed roots were the bones of the long dead.

THE POISON

Yew is stuck in grief and cannot imagine ever being joyful again. Long ago they lost something or someone dear to them and it colours every aspect of their life. They are mired in their sorrow, which has become like a pair of comfortable old shoes. They feel they can never be happy again and cannot accept the changes the loss has brought them. In their darkest moments they feel that no one else has suffered as much as them, that they have suffered the most.

THE ANTIDOTE

One thing people can always rely on is change, because life is in constant flux and can transform in an instant. From a limited perspective our human part detests change and will do anything to maintain the status quo, but resistance is futile: life will change as we grow. Yew will enjoy gains and suffer losses, and the more they can accept this as part of life on earth the more they will enjoy the crazy ride. They can set down the heavy load of being a hapless victim beholden to fate by embracing change, realising that everything is just as it should be. As Apollinaire said: 'After each sorrow, joy came back again.'

36. Liberty Cap
Surrender

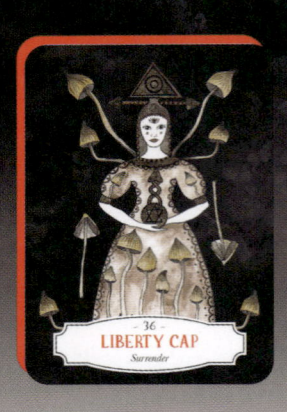

Botanical name: Psilocybe semilanceata.
Energy: magickal, hidden and mysterious.
Other names: magic mushroom, blue legs, pixie caps, witches' hats.
Traditional/medicinal uses: promising studies show their use in micro-dose amounts combats depression, addiction and anxiety.
Magickal/historical uses: this magic mushroom contains the hallucinogenic substance psilocybin and is associated with super consciousness, fairies and elementals. It has been used in rituals since ancient times for prophetic visions and insights.

🍄 THE POISON 🍄

The disempowered Liberty Cap doesn't allow for intuition, pottering or time to dream because they want to achieve their human goals as quickly as possible. They will never give in and never give up and will keep knocking on closed doors. They have decided what their life plan is, and there is no deviating from their rigid schedule: they must stick to this plan! There is a logical progression of things to cross off their to-do list so they can be seen as successful. They are locked in their own minds, trying to use willpower and force to create things and not allowing for creativity, insight or new experiences.

THE ANTIDOTE

Liberty must realise that the universe has a plan for them that may not fit their inflexible ideas about how their life should pan out. An empowered Liberty surrenders and lets go, allowing their higher self to be in charge. They may go on many magical side adventures and might not achieve their goals as quickly as they would like, but they must trust that what is meant for them will come to them. As Lao Tzu said: 'By letting go it all gets done. The world is won by those that let it go. But if you try and try the world is beyond the winning.'

Bibliography

Bonnet, M.S. and Basson, P.W., 2004, The toxicology of *Amarita virosa*: the destroying angel, https://pubmed.ncbi.nlm.nih.gov/15532702, accessed 17 March 2023.

Demir, Nazan, Daşdemir, Sila Nezahat, Kaplan, Alevcan and Demir, Yaşar, 2022, 'Determination of some bioactivities of *Convallaria majalis* L. (lily of the valley); isolation pharmaceutical active ingredient and investigation into its industrial usage', *Middle East Journal of Science*, doi.org/10.51477/mejs.1196088, accessed 17 March 2023.

Department for International Trade, 2019, Welsh-grown daffodils help tackle Alzheimer's, London, UK, https://www.gov.uk/government/news/welsh-grown-daffodils-help-tackle-alzheimers, accessed 17 March 2023.

Fatal death cap mushroom may ultimately be a life-saver, 2018, https://vancouversun.com/news/local-news/fatal-death-cap-mushroom-may-ultimately-be-a-life-saver, accessed 17 March 2023.

Feeney, Kevin, 2020, Fly Agaric as Medicine: From Traditional to Modern Use, 2020, https://www.researchgate.net/publication/345154633_Fly_Agaric_as_Medicine_From_Traditional_to_Modern_Use, accessed 17 March 2023.

Feeney, Kevin, 2022, Fly Agaric: A Compendium of History, Pharmacology, Mythology, and Exploration, https://chacruna.net/fly-agaric-amanita-muscaria-traditional-modern-therapeutic-uses, accessed 17 March 2023.

Grieve, M. (nd), Bryony, Black, https://botanical.com/botanical/mgmh/b/brybla75.html, accessed 17 March 2023.

Grieve, M. (nd), Lily, Madonna, https://botanical.com/botanical/mgmh/l/lilmad24.html, accessed 17 March 2023.

Grieve, M. (nd), Mistletoe, https://botanical.com/botanical/mgmh/m/mistle40.html, accessed 17 March 2023.

Grieve, M. (nd), Thornapple, https://botanical.com/botanical/mgmh/t/thorna12.html, accessed 17 March 2023.

Heinrich, Michael and Lee Teoh, Hooi, 2004, 'Galanthamine from snowdrop – the development of a modern drug against Alzheimer's disease from local Caucasian knowledge', *Journal of Ethnopharmacology*, 92(2–3), pp. 147–62, https://pubmed.ncbi.nlm.nih.gov/15137996, accessed 17 March 2023.

Heritage Garden (nd), Calla lily (*Zantedeschia aethiopica*), http://heritagegarden.uic.edu/calla-lily-zantedeschia-aethiopica, accessed 17 March 2023.

Khatri, Dharmendra Kumar and Juvekar, Archana Ramesh, 2015, 'Propensity of *Hyoscyamus niger* seeds methanolic extract to allay stereotaxically rotenone-induced Parkinson's disease symptoms in rats', *Oriental Pharmacy and Experimental Medicine*, 15(4), pp. 327–39, https://doi.org/10.1007/s13596-015-0202-x, accessed 17 March 2023.

Michael, Coby, 2021, The *Poison Path Herbal: Baneful Herbs, Medicinal Nightshades, and Ritual Entheogens*, Inner Traditions/Bear, Rochester, Vermont.

Potterton, David (ed.), 1997, *Culpeper's Colour Herbal*, Clippenham, Foulsham, UK.

Sample, Ian, 2022, Magic mushrooms' psilocybin can alleviate severe depression when used with therapy, https://www.theguardian.com/science/2022/nov/02/magic-mushrooms-psilocybin-alleviate-severe-depression-alongside-therapy, accessed 17 March 2023.

Stewart, Amy, 2010, *Wicked Plants: the A-Z of plants that kill, maim, intoxicate and otherwise*, Timber Press, Portland, Oregon.

WebMD (nd), Foxglove – Uses, Side Effects, and More, https://www.webmd.com/vitamins/ai/ingredientmono-287/foxglove, accessed 17 March 2023.

WildFoodUK (nd), Hemlock Water Dropwort, 2019, https://www.wildfooduk.com/edible-wild-plants/hemlock-water-dropwort, accessed 17 March 2023.

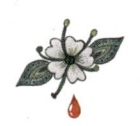

Acknowledgements

I'd like to thank the following people for inspiration:

The teachings of Suzanne Giesemann and
The Awakened Way,
suzannegiesemann.com/the-awakened-way

The teachings of Dolores Cannon,
dolorescannon.com

The teachings of Nanci L. Danison,
nancidanison.com

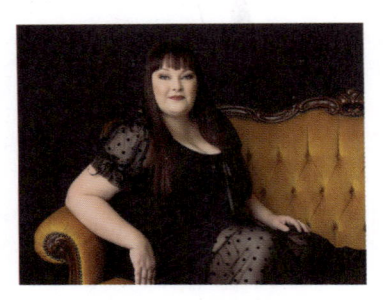

ABOUT THE AUTHOR AND ILLUSTRATOR

Priestess Moon's oracle cards are divination tools designed to help you access your intuition. Using the cards will support you in answering questions and taking action and will reassure you and bring solace. She paints magickal energy into the artworks and writes the guidebook based on life experiences, metaphysical concepts and extensive research.

Priestess Moon is the author of *Enchanted Spell Oracle*, *Making Magick*, *Making Magick Oracle* and *Enchanted Unicorn Oracle*. Her oracle decks come from the heart and are created with the wish that they bring you joy, delight and comfort.

Website: priestessmoondesign.com
Instagram: priestessmoondesign
Facebook: priestess.moon99
YouTube: priestessmoondesign